DRIVE AWAY
DISEASES

DR. GOMATIRAMAN

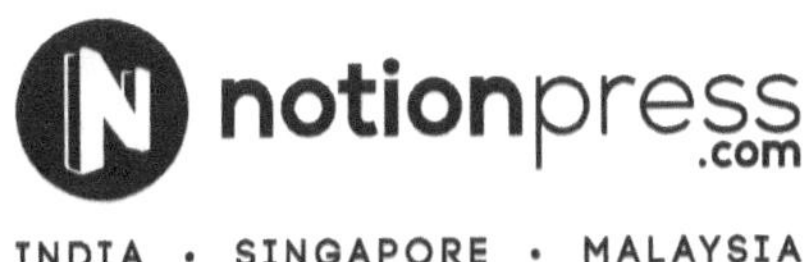

Notion Press Media Pvt Ltd

No. 50, Chettiyar Agaram Main Road,
Vanagaram, Chennai, Tamil Nadu – 600 095

First Published by Notion Press 2021
Copyright © Dr. Gomatiraman 2021
All Rights Reserved.

ISBN 978-1-63940-325-7

AUTHOR'S APPEAL

Dear Readers,

Blessings to all.

I always believe "Health is wealth". If a person is healthy he will be able to enjoy his life. If the health is disturbed everything gets disturbed. Therefore it is necessary to follow certain discipline to keep ourselves healthy. I was personally guiding people to keep away from diseases and almost all those who practiced were successful in maintaining healthy life.

Today we are under the influence of Covid, a pandemic disease that is eating up millions of life everyday and brought the human life to stand still. This pandemic has created great fear in the minds of people and destroyed the love for the fellow beings.

Schools, colleges, business, charitable organisations are close down. Only Hospitals and medical shops are opened. There is no place for funeral for burial. People are afraid to collect the dead bodies of their own family members if they happen to die due to Covid.

Everyone is giving their ideas to get rid of Covid in the form of different medicines that are known to them without having proper knowledge of the disease or knowing the need of individual human body.

I felt that it is my duty to guide the people by giving knowledge to keep them away from any disease so that we can create a healthy society. Therefore I am trying to put forth my ideas in a simple and easy way so that it can help the humanity to drive away the pandemic and epidemic diseases in future.

I will be happy if the reader could practice whatever is suggested over here and I am sure that you will be able to not only get rid of Covid but also protect yourself from any diseases.

Dr. GOMATIRAMAN

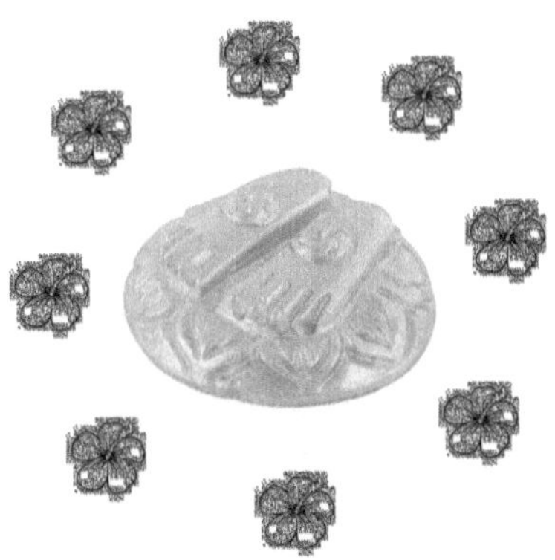

I DEDICATE THIS BOOK AT THE LOTUS FEET

OF

THE MOTHER, SRI AUROBINDO ASHRAM,
POINDICHERRY.

LET THE MOTHER'S BLESSINGS BE BESTOWED

ON

EVERYONE WHO READ THIS BOOK

AND

HELP THEM TO MANIFEST THE DIVINE IN
THEM.

I THANK THE MOTHER FOR HER BLESSINGS ON
ME.

DR.GOMATIRAMAN

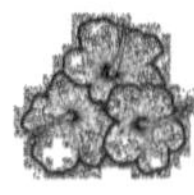
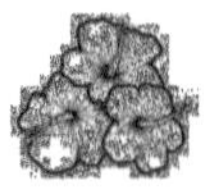
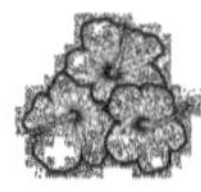
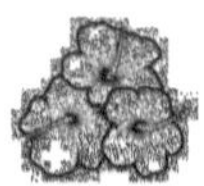

CONTENTS

INTRODUCTION

Everyone wants to lead a happy life. Happiness in life is possible only e if a person is healthy and do not suffer from any disease. Whenever a person fall sick immediately he/she look for medicine are rush to the doctor for solution. How nice it would be if you are able to live a life without attack of any disease!

In this book I am attempting to guide the people to get rid of diseases and protect themselves from the attack of diseases well in advance so that you never fall sick at all. These are easy methods that do not cost you any money, medicine or even the support of doctor.

You can practice these methods on your bed, while walking and while travelling. Just change in your thoughts, in your attitudes and your approach can keep you away from the diseases.

These methods are already practiced by various people and they were able to come out of even chronic illnesses.

It is not compulsory that you have to practice all methods given in the book but you can try whichever method suits you or brings success in driving away the diseases.

DISEASE

What is disease? When your ease is disturbed you feel disturbance in your easy life. In other words dis + ease = disease. Disturbance in ease is disease. Disease can be physical or mental. When you lose your balance in your body that becomes physical disease and when you lose your mental strength that becomes mental disease. Physical and mental health is equally important for a peaceful life.

Diseases do not attack you directly. First it comes into your environment and then touches your body and thereafter it enters into your system and put you on the bed. If you are able to identify the disease when it enters into environment, and reject that thought, you can easily reject the diseases from attacking you. For that you must know your body, its responses, its belief and its need. You should also have an idea about your mental setup regarding any disease.

For example, sometime you could have felt that you may get fever or you may get headache. Ultimately you start feeling feverish or headache after an hour or two. When you felt that you may get feverish or headache the disease entered into your environment. Then, when you accepted that thought it touched your body and entered into your system. The result is that you got fever or headache. At the time of feeling feverish or headache if you are able to reject that thought, the disease will not be able to get in your environment or enter into your body. For this you have to you simply divert your mind and involve yourself into some positive activities that can keep you happy. Having no response from your end the thought has to get away from your environment and you are protected from falling sick.

KNOW THE SOURCE OF DISEASE

Whenever you fall sick, take 10 or 15 minutes to think as to why you feel sick, recollect the similar disturbance you had in your health in the past. You will come out with various reasons such as – where you went, what you did, to whom you met, what you ate etc. etc. Identify and compare the reasons for the illness if it were repeated again and again. Try to remember as to how many times you were responsible to get the same illness. If the illness is repeated several times you have to identify what was wrong from your part to get the illness. Similarly list the situations where you had successfully handled and came out of any illness whether it was small or big and those incidents where you were not able to find a solution. You need not devote special time for this. You can do this at anytime when you are alone. Simply you should be aware of your thoughts, words and action and understand what kind of thoughts/words/actions make you dull.

Positive and negative thoughts are moving in the atmosphere. Similarly germs and bacteria are also prevailing in the atmosphere. They enter into your environment when you have the receptivity for a particular thought, vibration etc.

This can be explained in a very simple way. Whenever you happen to visit a patient in the hospital, you feel sad to look at the condition of the patient. Why? It is because the patient and the family members of the patient are sad. When you enter into a sad atmosphere, naturally you also get influenced by the sadness. It means that you have the receptivity for the sadness prevailing in the environment and that is why the sadness could enter into you and make you feel sorry for the patient. Whereas when the patient goes to the doctor, the Doctor is very neutral because he is not having the receptivity of the sadness but his intention is to identify the condition of the patient. Therefore he does not get influenced by the sadness but he is able to look at the real condition of the patient and give him necessary treatment.

If you happen to visit any patient in the hospital or in home, please remember that you do not discuss about the dangers of the disease or about the dangers that others had undergone to the patient or to their family members. These kinds of discussions will increase the fear in them and the patient will take long time to get cured. On the other hand you can encourage the patient to keep faith, wish him speedy recovery that would help the patient to recover soon.

Pandemic and epidemic diseases spread fast because of the fear that is being established by the people around us. The fear of getting attacked makes the people to become over cautious and ultimately make them victim to the attack of the pandemic or epidemic diseases. Instead of creating fear in the people if the if we could convey the message in the form of alertness, awareness and remedial measures that would help to drive away the Pandemic & Epidemic diseases from spreading.

THOUGHT FORCE

Thought plays an important role in human beings life. If you are able to understand the power of thought, you will be able to get rid of so many difficulties in life. Whatever you think that is sent on the air. Then the thought starts its work to convert it into reality. It does not retire without converting itself in to reality. Sometime you think of someone very deeply for some time. When you get some other work, you forget the previous thought and engage in your new work. But this thought works out and brings the person before you in a situation where you feel awkward to interact.

For example; Let us assume that sitting in your home, you think about a person who cheated you and went far away from you. Suddenly the thought of the person came in your mind. You plan in your mind as to how you will react if he appears suddenly before you. This thought moves in the air and creates a link between you and the person. Depending on the intensity of your thought, the connection between you two gets established soon or later. Suddenly this person appears before you and you could not do anything according to the plan you made in your mind. The thought you sent in the air had done its duty by bringing the person before you in the way you wanted him to appear before you. Since you travelled a long way from that thought, when it gets materialized it creates disturbances instead giving happiness. Any thought sent in the air moves around and dissolves after its materialization. Therefore it is necessary to have awareness about your thoughts always.

Most of the diseases are able to enter in our body because of our thoughts only. Our subconscious mind stores all our experience and reflects it from time to time according to the situation. Repeated diseases attacking us on a particular season or on a particular situation is the result of our experience only. If you are able to consider the disease like a passing cloud, it would not come back again. For example; if you happen to get wet in the rain, you have the fear that you may get cold or fever; if you are forced to move around in the sunlight, you feel that you may get headache; if you happen to eat some spicy items in any party or function, you feel that you make get acidity. The previous experiences you had, had been recorded in your subconscious mind so strongly that you quite naturally decide that you will be getting the particular problem in your health if you happened to expose yourself to a given situation.

The remedy for this problem is very simple. Never come to a conclusion that you will fall sick if you do such and such things. On the other hand you try to develop a faith in you that this discomfort will get away from your body and you will never be disturbed by it again.

If you observe your thoughts you will find that most of the time your negative thoughts become responsible to create sufferings in your life. You always have preconceived idea that this may cause this problem, and that problem happens in real life. For example; if your teenage daughter did not come back from school in time you start thinking all kind of negative things. This thought goes in the air and create a situation for her to get into to difficulties. Suddenly one fine day you find what you feared that had happened.

You will be able to get rid of almost all the diseases, if you are able to develop positive thoughts in yourself as well as for your beloved ones. Your self confidence will boost the immunity in you and it will bring all positive things in your life. Having a strong thought that "you are healthy; that no disease can attack you; you are healthy; the people in your home are also healthy" will bring a positive atmosphere in your home and diseases cannot enter into your environment.

Following examples can give clear ideas about our preconceived ideas and experiences that put you into to illness or are any difficulties.

- Let us assume that you keep fasting on a particular day in every month. That day you will never feel tired or feel the need of eating food. It is because your subconscious mind had understood that on this particular day I will not be getting the food and this acceptance helps you to get rid of hunger.

Similarly if you happen to miss your breakfast or lunch due to external pressure you feel tired and you want to take rest. This is because your subconscious mind feels that you didn't take your breakfast and your stomach is empty therefore you have no energy to continue any work.

This clearly shows that it is your thought of missing something are giving up something that brings changes in our body and you start feeling energetic or tired.

- Whenever you return from long travel you catch hold of cough and cold you will get cough and cold. This is because of your preconceived idea that you will get cold and cough if you go for long travelling. In case you are able to identify that it is your preconceived idea that is bringing you the diseases, you will definitely reject such thoughts and protect yourself from the regular disease that is attacking you after travelling. The same thing goes well for all the diseases. Whenever any disease attacks you and a particular time or after a particular work or in a particular season you can understand this happens because of your preconceived ideas.

- When you happen to go to a marriage ceremony or a birthday party you will be carrying with you the positive thoughts of the person in whose function you are going to participate.

You will naturally get a positive feeling and after entering into that atmosphere you get influenced by the environment and you enjoy being with them. When you return home you carry with you the happiness that you gained from the atmosphere.

Similarly if you have to attend a funeral rite, you carry the memory of the person who passed away and feel sad for missing him/her. When you return home you carry along with you the sadness that leads you to depression naturally. This is the influence of the environment that brings energy or depression in your life.

When you feel happy, you feel energetic and when you fall in to depression, you start feeling sick. Repeated depression may make you feel down and may lead you to serious illness.

If you are able to understand the reason for your illness, you will reject such thoughts that cannot help you and encourage only those thoughts that will help you to gain energy and be creative.

- You are in search for a job. You attended several interviews. You found that you are being rejected for some or other reasons. This led you to frustration and you fall victim to drugs to escape from the failure. Your weakness turns into addiction and you become victim to diseases.

In case you take little time to find out and understand as to why you are being rejected every time and try to improve your quality according to the demand of the employer or market or try to choose a job that suits your character and ability, you will get selected and can lead a happy life. If you are able to learn this trick that can bring out of any difficulties you would never fall sick or fall into depression or allow weakness to make you feel sick.

- In your office environment if you find your bosses or superior or your colleagues does not co-operate with you, you get irritated and start hating the job that you are doing. Sometime you leave the job and sit idle at home or join some other job that is worst than what you were doing earlier. Repeated change in the job and repeated occurrence of disturbances, non recognition and partiality also leads to depression. Every time you fall into depression there is a physical change inside that forms the foundation for blood pressure, diabetes, fear and dullness in your life.

- You should also understand that your behaviour and your mood reflect on the behaviour of your family members. The life becomes hell for such a person who is unable to understand the situation and people around him. He is not happy in his office as he expects his superiors to understand him. He is not happy in his home because his family members do not understand him. He wants to escape or get away from all these people and environment. These kind of escapism or running away from the fact leads a person to wrong companionship and he becomes the victim of bad habits like smoking, tobacco, consuming alcohol, womanizing etc. All these drug addictions form the base for ill health to attack in future permanently.

One thing you have to understand is that changing yourself is in your hands but changing others is not in your reach. It is better to identify your strengths and weaknesses, use your strength properly and give up the weaknesses.

You can't expect others to behave the way you expect them to do, especially when you are under the obligation of your employer or superior. It is you who has to change yourself and cannot expect the management to change. If you are able to understand this fact, you will never get caught in the situational influences and will able to overcome from any kind of depression.

- Sometimes the negative opinions of the people about your health also cause illness. Your family members would have experienced that if you take cold water bath, you may get cold or if you drink ice water you may get throat infection, if you eat a particular food you may get certain problems in your health. Such kind of opinions of others especially of your near and dears also put you in to ill health. In some cases the unwanted worries of the over protective parents put their children into ill health. They possess a kind of fear in them that their child may get affected if they are exposed to rain or sunlight etc. Such worries also bring in diseases in the children. Though maintaining discipline in everything is necessary in life, it should not come in the way of the health of the children.

- Parents should bring up their children in such a way they should learn to be positive enough to overcome if they fall sick. Children naturally possess such capability in them, but the parents discourage them and create fear in them and the children become weak to come out of illness. Children should be trained to be in friendly with the nature. They should also encourage positive thoughts in the children and prepare them to manage any imbalance caused in the body.

We can avoid depression and diseases if we are able to understand our thoughts, our preconceived ideas, our judgement on the people with whom we are associated, our companionship, neighbourhood, relationships and bring positive changes in our thoughts and ideas. Our problem is that we do everything mechanically. We are not conscious as to what we are saying, how we are reacting, why we are doing a particular thing etc. If we become conscious of our speech and every action at any given situation, we will be able to understand those things that go without our control.

If you want to live a disease free life then you must be conscious on everything that you do. You don't need medicine; you don't need to do any diet; simply understanding what should be the right action or attitude that you have to take at a particular point of time. Initially it may be difficult to apply this at every level because of your mechanical life; but if you persist, definitely you can reduce the moment of disturbances and diseases, you can keep yourself happy you can keep the people associated with you happy. This is the will power that makes the negative forces to think thousand times before entering your environment.

You must take care that negative thoughts like fear, confusion, anger, hatred kinds of qualities does not enter your environment. Now let us understand how negative qualities or bringing diseases in our life.

Anger increases blood pressure, leads us to heart attack; sometime even to death. Fear stops our progress, make us week and create confusion sometime gives great shock that may cause death. Confusion always delays the decision making process. It creates misunderstanding and hatred for others.

Hatred should be considered as a dangerous disease because it is worst than poison. Explaining a natural incident that had happened in one of my neighbour's house would be appropriate to explain the power of hatred.

I was conducting sat sangh every Sunday in my home. One day a lady named Mythili around 45 years of age came to my house. I was in the first floor. She climbed the stairs and reached my home. She was finding it difficult to breath. I gave her a glass of water. She said water will not help her because according to the doctor she is having a hole in her heart and she is about to live only for another three months only. I asked her who all are there in her family. She replied that she has a son, an arrogant and ignorant daughter-in-law named Vasanti and a grandson. The narration that she had given about her daughter in law made me feel that this lady totally hates her daughter-in-law Vasanti. I asked her whether she is sure that she will die in three months time. She said "yes". Then I asked her, will she be happy if Vasanti becomes happy after her death. Mythili said, "No".

I suggested her why can't she try to forgive Vasanti and give her love so that Vasanti will feel sad for abusing her mother in law Mythili if she dies. Mythili thought for a while and, she nodded her head and proceeded to her home. On the way she found a flower seller selling jasmine flower. She stopped him and bought some flowers and reached home. She gave the flowers to Vasanti and inquired whether she had the lunch or not. Vasanti was surprised on this question and she said "not yet" and she kept the flowers in front of the Gods photograph. Mythili ordered Vasanti to bring the food so that they can have the lunch together. Listening to this Vasanti felt so emotional; tears rolled down on her cheeks. Mythili scolded her and told her to stop crying and serve the food. When they sat for lunch, for the first time Mythili took the initiative and served the food to both. Again the emotional situation increased. In the evening Mythili made Vasanti to sit in front of her and combed her hair. She asked her to bring the flowers and clipped the flower on her hair. Vasanti fell at the feet of Mythili and expressed her gratitude for the love. Mythili also felt emotional and the hatred disappeared forever. After few days when the medicines for the mother-in-law got exhausted, Vasanti attempted to buy the medicines; but Mythili refused by saying "I have only limited time. Why to waste money on me. No need of buying medicine. Let the lord decide my destiny."

Mythili came to me after around six months. I inquired about her health. From her I came to know that she stopped taking the medicine long back. She also confessed that her daughter-in-law Vasanti was a very good girl and Mythili could not understand her feelings. She confirmed that she is very happy now and she is not taking medicine also. I reminded her that it is already six months over. The Doctor had given only three months time and the three months had already elapsed. I suggested her to go to the hospital and have a check-up once again. She accepted my suggestion and went to the hospital and had a check-up. Doctors were surprised to note that there is no symptom of hole in her heart. There was no trace of any operation too. She came back and showed me the report. She lived for another 20 years happily with her son, daughter in law and grandson.

This was a great learning for me that hatred can make hole in the heart and love can even cure a hole in the heart without medicine. I am sure that this real incident will make you think where all you are wrong and responsible for your own difficulties and diseases.

There is also another story about Saint Jamadagni and his wife Renuka Devi. Both of them were living a saintly life. Their thoughts, feelings, environment and everything were so pure there was no place for any negativity over there.

Everyday Renuka Devi used to go to the nearby river early in the morning, take bath and make a pot from the river sand, fill the pot with the river water and offer the same for performing the religious rites that the Saint Jamadagni used to do.

One day when Renuka Devi bowed to take a dip in the river, she found the shadow of a Gandharva (An angel) in the water. For a moment she exclaimed how beautiful is he and she looked up on the sky. Then she took her bath and attempted to make the pot from the sand as usual; but she was unable to make the pot from the sand even after trying for hours together. Saint Jamadagni was worried and tried to find the situation with the help of his insight and found that his wife had lost her purity as she admired another man in her life.

Saint Jamadagni had five sons. He called them and ordered them to cut off the head of Renuka Devi as she failed to maintain her purity as a wife. Only Parshuram his youngest son came forward to obey the order of his father. He met his mother and asked her for apology as he is going to cut off her head to obey the order of the father. He cut her head off and threw it away at the river shore and reported the fact to the father. The father was very happy to see the obedience of his son and asked him to ask for any boon that he wishes.

Parshuram asked that he wants his mother back. Saint Jamadagni was further happy to know the intelligence of his son. He gave him some holy water and advised Parshuram to fix the head with the body and sprinkle the holy water on his mother and she will turn alive. When Parshuram went to the river shore with the holy water to bring back his mother alive, he found there were two bodies and two heads lying on the river shore. He came to know that a prostitute of a local area was also punished to death and her body was also thrown at the river shore. Therefore there were two bodies and two heads.

Parshuram was familiar with his mother's face but not with the body because he always looked at his mother's face and spoke. Unable to identify the body of the mother, Parshuram thought that he will give life to his mother as well as to the prostitute. He fixed the heads with the body sprinkled the holy water on them. Both the women became alive. Now the mother said, "Parshuram, what did you do? You fixed my head with the prostitute's body. How can I live in this impure body? I can't go back to your father also. This is the punishment for me for allowing the impure thought to enter in me even for a while." Unable to go back to her husband, she left to a lonely place with the view to spend her remaining life in doing penance.

The moral of the story is that a moment of negative thought had ruined the entire saintly life of Renuka and she had to live in a body of a prostitute for the rest of her life.

If we have to face the consequences of our thoughts with such immediate effects what will be our destiny and how will be our life which we have to just think.

REMEDIES

Now let us discuss some remedial measures to get rid of diseases. One of the best ways to drive away disease is "Auto Positive Suggestion". You had already seen that it is your negative thoughts that bring you diseases. So it is necessary to develop positive thoughts in you so that the negative effect does not come in your life. Auto Positive Suggestion is the best method through which the negative thoughts and feelings can be changed into positive thoughts and feelings.

AUTO POSITIVE SUGGESTION

Auto positive suggestion is an art of speaking to one's own self. You can speak to your body that it is healthy and it will not allow any disease to get into it. You can also speak to your mind that you are healthy and it is not necessary every time you get some symptom and you get the disease simultaneously. Auto Positive Suggestion is a practice to talk to the body and mind whenever negative thoughts get into you or whenever you feel weak or depressed or frustrated.

If you feel tired, you have to suggest yourself that you are energetic and divert your mind in some creative or very interesting activity. You will be surprised to see the result that you become energetic in few minutes.

Similarly when you feel depressed, find the reason for the depression and then suggest to your mind that the depression is not going to help you in anyway. Repeatedly suggesting the mind that you don't need the depression, will force the depression to get away from your environment.

When you get angry, try to tell yourself, "I am cool. I am normal". Instead of expressing your anger immediately without awareness, if you suggest to you to remain cool and calm, the power of anger will go down and the consequences of your anger will be reduced considerably.

The first thing you have to do is to be aware of the attack of anger, depression frustration, hatred etc. Once you become aware of the negative qualities and its consequences that you had to face later, you will definitely be able to develop the habit of Auto Positive Suggestion that would help you to protect your body and your mind and keep you away from the attack of any disease.

Whenever you feel an indication of any disease, you have to tell to yourself that you are healthy and no disease can attack you. You have to tell this with total confident and power that the thought of getting the disease has to get away from you. It is just like closing the door of your house to a stranger without any mercy, so that he goes away from your door. You can repeat the statement that you are healthy as long as you feel the symptom. If you have decided not to allow the disease to enter in to your body and suggest your body that you are healthy, the body will reject the symptom of the illness and you will be protected from the attack of the disease.

Normally, when someone doesn't obey your order, anger pops in; when things do not go according to your expectation, you get frustrated; when someone cheats you to whom you trusted the most, the disappointment enters in you; when you listen to any rumour about the happening around you, the fear gets in you. All these things happen quite naturally and mechanically because of your habits and preconceived ideas.

If you want the Auto Positive Suggestion to be successful to bring changes in you, you have to become aware as to what all the situations during which you fall victim to negative qualities. Then you have to be aware before reacting to such situations. It may take little time but it will help you in the long run.

Let us understand this with an example. Assume that you happened to wet in the rain. You already had the experience that if you remain wet for a longer time, you get cold and fever. Now the fear comes into you that you may get cold and fever because you got wet in the rain; ultimately you permitted the cold & fever into you and you need to go the doctor for medicine. Now what you have to do is to suggest yourself, "I am healthy. I will not get cold or fever. I am totally healthy". Whenever you get the symptoms of cold, cough or fever you must repeat the above sentences as many times as possible. The more is the power of your feeling the fastest will be the relief.

Following are some real experiences of my students of Somaiya College, Mumbai, who had experienced when they practiced Auto Positive Suggestion in their life to come out of their weaknesses.

Experience No.1

Vidya was in 10th standard. She was an average student. She was put in to stress by her class teacher, her parents and tuition teacher that Board exam is very tough and she has to study day and night to get through the examination. She was weak in English & Mathematics and it was bothering her a lot.

She was advised to observe her thoughts and note down the same. While noting down, she herself understood that she is studying well, but the stress from teachers and parents made her feel afraid. She was suggested to promise the parents and teachers that she is studying well and she would get through with high percentage in the Board exam. She was also asked to speak to herself that she has no fear because she is preparing well for the exam. She did this practice for about 10 days and scored above 60% in all subjects including English & Mathematics.

Experience No.2

Raju was a college student and he was the only son to his parents. His mother used to be worried all the time about him. Whenever she reads any negative news about the youth or see any such things on Television, she used to imagine that her son is also getting involved in such activities like smoking, consuming alcohol etc. When he returns home, he used to ask him to blow his mouth and become relaxed when he had not consumed alcohol etc.

One day Raju was forced to consume alcohol when he went to attend his friend's birthday party. When all his friends were taking the drink, he could not say "No" and had returned home duly drunk. Raju's mother was shocked that her fear became true. Slowly he became addict to smoking and alcohol. When his habit became a great disturbance in the family, the mother came to the college for counselling from the professors and to find solution.

She was informed that she has to give up her fear and think positive about her son because incidents that are displayed on the TV are simply for excitement. It is not real. People who do such acting do it to earn money. She was not willing to agree that her negative thoughts can change the life of her own son and she was arguing that as a mother she had all the right to worry about her son and expect that he does not get in to any bad habits. After much persuasion she agreed to observe her thoughts about her son and whenever she gets a negative thought, think positive about him and visualize that he is changed and gave up the company of bad friends and concentrating on his studies. Though she did not fully happy with our counseling that this method would work, she tried and started the practice. On the first day itself she found that he came home without drinking. She was so happy and started following the **"Auto Positive Suggestion"** seriously. In three months time, Raju got rid of all his bad companions and started concentrating on his studies.

Experience No.3

Mohan was 22 years old and was in search of employment for more than two years. Whenever he went for interview, he was nervous. He had a fear that he may not get selected. And he did not get selected anywhere and he was highly frustrated. He started losing his confidence and stopped trying for any more jobs. Parents started criticizing him for sitting idle and every day there was fight at home on this issue.

He came with his mother for Counseling. While discussing it was found that he went to attend the first interview with lots of hope. But he was not able to answer the questions properly at the interview due to fear. The fear was so strong that he attended all the interviews without confident. He was explained that he should prepare well for the interview and should be bold in answering. He was made to understand that interview is nothing but a conversation between the employer and the candidate. If the candidate is able to convince the employer, it is for sure that he would get the job. He was suggested that he should think positive and attend the interview with confidence. He tried to have positive thoughts and used the method of **"Auto Positive Suggestion"** and got selected in the next interview.

There are several experiences people had gained by practicing Auto Positive Suggestion method. Instead of filling the pages with the experiences, I wish that the reader should try to practice Auto Positive Suggestion to come out of their difficulties; so that it would be your authenticated experience which may help you to help others to develop positive vibration around them.

In today's condition we are suffering not only from noise pollution, environmental pollution etc., but also the thought pollution that is taking away the life of human beings. People's minds are filled with fear and rumours to such extent that the entire universe is polluted with negative thoughts and negative feelings. There are only few people who are trying to be positive and asking others to be positive. Unless each one understands it is me, my thoughts and my vibrations are bringing positive or negative things in my life, it is difficult to drive away diseases.

FITNESS

Next is the requirement of physical fitness to keep away from diseases. You had already learnt that the imbalance or a disturbance in the equilibrium in the body cause the diseases. In other words, the body indicates when there is disturbance in its function. If we understand the indication and set right the issue, the disease disappears. If you want to drive away the diseases then you need to maintain physical fitness, mental fitness and emotional balance.

During 18th and 19th century technology was not that much advanced compared to today's live. Advancement in technology brought so many changes in human life. All the manual works are being done with the use of machines. In Olden times people did all the work by themselves, they had all kinds of physical movements, muscle movements that helped them to maintain proper health.

Man used to go to the paddy field, work under the sun, stand in the water for hours together, carry heavy loads on the shoulder or keeping them in the cart and pulling them the entire weight, used to travel long distances by walk or used bicycle to go anywhere. These kinds of activities helped them in muscle movements of all parts of the body. They lived with the nature. They ate homemade food. They lived in joint family and each member of the family shared the responsibilities. So the amount of stress was less; their work made them strong; their coordination with the nature prevented them from diseases.

Similarly the women at home also performed such activities that naturally made them to do physical exercises. They pulled water from the well, ground the spices on the stone; bent themselves to sweep the room and mop the rooms; dusting the wall; they used to prepare food by using firewood stove; they had to blow air to make the firewood burn; they walked down to the river or nearby pond to take bath. Washing the clothes of all the family members also was the duties of the women at home.

Less furniture was used in the home. Guests used to sit on the mat provided to them. Family members sat on the ground to eat their food and they had the practice sleep on the floor. All these practices helped them to maintain proper health and protected them from the attack of epidemic or pandemic diseases.

Unfortunately in today's condition the advancement of Technology changed the lifestyle of the human beings. Cooking is done on the gas stove in standing posture. The woman stands for hours together to do the cooking. Then they sit on the Sofa or chair; sleep on the bed; grind in the mixture and grinder; bath under the shower and wash the clothes in the washing machine. The entire body weight is loaded on the knee when a person stands in a particular posture for hours together. This results in the knee pain. Not having enough hip movement or muscle movement blocks the blood circulation in the body and ultimately creates back pain, neck pain etc. Junk food creates acidity and indigestion.

Similarly in the case of men, they prefer to use petrol vehicles to go fast; rash driving results in accidents and sometime causing the life. This also spread pollution in the environment; they work in the office by sitting in a particular posture for hours together; Attraction towards white collar job resulted in less agriculture production and ultimately the prices and demand of the food products increased.

It may not be possible for the present day generation to go back to 18th 19th century life, but if they are able to develop awareness in them about the necessity of physical fitness and follow the easy methods given below to remain healthy forever will highly help them to get rid of diseases.

If you are physically fit, when you happen to walk under the hot sun, you will not faint; similarly when you get wet in the rain, you will not catch cold or cough; if there is any spreading disease like malaria etc. your body will produce the immunity to reject the entry of such diseases and keep you protected; if you happen to work for longer hours, your body would produce enough energy to complete the task; if you don't get food for one time, your body would have the capacity to manage without the food. If you possess such a flexible and strong body, you can say that you are physically fit.

Such strength, flexibility and immunity come from physical discipline. It should start right from the childhood. Your food habits and food timings should be standard. You should always eat healthy food and reject junk food. Junk food may be tasty and easy to buy and eat, but that ruins your health. Do not overeat for the sake of taste. Eat only to the need. The quantity of food should be 50%, water 25% and the stomach should be kept 25% empty. If you eat this way, the food would easily get mixed in the water and there would be enough space in the stomach for grinding and the food would get easily digested. Once you take your breakfast, meal or dinner you should walk for a while, so that it helps in digesting. You should also give enough time between meals; the amount of food for breakfast and lunch can be more but at dinner, the food that you eat should be light; because after dinner you go to sleep and there is no physical activity for your body. If you take heavy dinner, you will add cholesterol to your body. You must drink more water during day time. If you drink minimum one litre water in the morning in empty stomach, you will not have constipation problem; you need not go for any dieting to reduce your weight.

Fitness of the body can be maintained by regular physical exercises, breathing exercises, maintaining regular food habits and by developing positive thoughts. Enough work to keep the body active, enough rest/sleep for regaining the energy is also must to gain a healthy body. Fitness in one area can strongly influence the fitness in other areas. For example, improving physical fitness enhances mental, emotional, and even spiritual activity.

Physical fitness is a state of health or the ability to perform the daily tasks without any difficulty. It could be gained by taking nutritious and timely food, regular physical exercise, maintaining hygienic and clean environment and proper sleep.

When the physical exercise is done regularly in the right way, with right intensity, duration and frequency, you can easily understand the improvement that takes place in your health. You will be able to perform your duty with energy and you will not feel fatigue at any point of time. You will be able to enjoy your life when you are physically fit.

Diet is also another important aspect to gain overall health and works the best in combination with physical exercise. Consuming balanced diet and doing regular physical exercises keeps you away from the doctor and medicines. If you understand the benefits of good health, you will understand the role of nutritious food and physical exercise that can keep you fresh and energetic.

Our heart needs enough amount of oxygen to pump the blood at regular rate without strain. Therefore, some exercises that helps to consume oxygen to be performed regularly. Physical health consists of many components. They are the key areas that should be taken care which are given below:

SOME SIMPLE WARMUP EXERCISES

Those who did not do exercise in the past, and now feel the need to do have to make their body flexible to make any movement can do the following exercises.

Lie on your back, raise your hands above your head and stretch as much as you can. Simultaneously stretch your legs downwards as much as you can.

Lie on your back; turn left; lift your right hand above the shoulder and stretch; bring it back to your thigh and stretch. Do the same by turning to right side;

Lie on your back; Lift your right leg to 90° and back; do the same with the left leg.

Lie on your back; rotate both your legs like cycling;

Lie on your stomach; lift your legs backward; lift your head upward and back to normal;

Stand straight, turn your head from left to right and right to left;

Stand straight; rotate your left hand in clockwise and anti clockwise; repeat the same with your right hand; thereafter rotate both the hands simultaneously;

Stand straight; try to touch your toes with your hands; initially don't strain much to touch the toes, but try maximum. If you regularly do this practice, you would be able to touch the toes in one week.

Stand straight; raise your right hand; let your right hand touch your right ears and bend left side by pulling the left hand along the thigh at left side, come back to normal position; repeat the same with left hand;

Keep both your hands on the hip, bend back ward to your maximum capability but without giving much stress to the muscles;

Do each of these practices for minimum five times. Once you experience that you can make these basic movements of your body easily, you can join some "Fitness/Yoga Class" to improve your Fitness.

Apart from the above exercises, you can also do jogging (running for a particular duration at a particular pace to a particular distance). This would help you to reduce your excess weight and proper digestion of food; those who cannot run, they can practice walking early in the morning at least for half an hour every day; those who have facilities or access can practice swimming. This helps to strengthen the arms and legs and helps the heart to function better. Riding in bicycle is also another type of activity that helps to strengthen the body.

People living in Metro cities face problems of space and time to do physical exercises. They can use the machine that helps to perform walking or running according to desired speed of the user. These machines help the people those who have knees and ankles pain.

Intake of nutritious food that is solid and fluid helps in proper digestion. Food that contains carbohydrates, proteins, fats, vitamins and minerals should be consumed according to the age and bodily requirement. Neither excess nor less should be consumed either out of taste or in the name of fasting. Consumption of quantity and frequency of food must be taken according to the individual need that the dietician decides. Proper food habits help in developing the immunity system of the body.

Balanced nutrition contains carbohydrates, proteins, fats, vitamins, minerals and water. These nutrients are available in grains, vegetables, fruits, milk products, meat and oil. The food that we eat and the water we drink must be clean and free from diseases. Eating proper amount of food at regular interval is must to maintain good health. Over eating, less eating, irregular eating, not eating are some of the serious issues that can be fatal.

Taking care of minor ailments with the homely remedy also helps to drive away diseases permanently. Avoid taking medicine for every little disturbance; try to tolerate pain for some time and use natural methods to get rid of pains. For example, if you get cold, try to inhale steam that would clear your cough; if you have fever, cover yourself with blanket and rest for a while; when you sweat, you will become alright. Fever is nothing but increase of temperature in your body; when the temperature is increased, the body throws it out; if you help the body by covering yourself with blanket, that would transfer into sweat and the body will come to normal temperature.

After the age of 30, reduce the quantity of salt, sugar & oil in your food; as we grow old, the capacity of the machines inside the body also become weak. Therefore, modification in the food habit is necessary to maintain a healthy body.

One should know when to consult the doctor. Taking medicines without the prescription of doctor will be dangerous. When the body gets disturbed it indicates the same in some kinds of pain. If we assume a headache is the pain in the head, we would be wrong. Headache may be due to eye-sight issue, over stress, non-digestion of food and so many other reasons. Therefore medicine should be taken only after consulting the Doctor.

Periodic rest and relaxation along with high quality sleep also helps to keep away from diseases. The brain and the body need sufficient rest and regular sleep to recover from the day to day stress experienced. To make the mind and body to function properly with fresh energy rest and relaxation is must. When the normal sleep gets disturbed the body and mind cannot get out of the daily stress and it makes the person to feel tired, function poorly, and he is easily exposed to diseases. Taking small nap after lunch helps the body to regain the energy. Any individual with normal health requires 7 to 9 hours sound sleep. The place where you sleep should be clean, calm, dark & with proper ventilation. It is also necessary to relax your mind before sleeping. Otherwise, the stress that you experienced during the day may come in the form of dream and you will feel drained away with energy. Therefore, try to listen to some light music, think something positive or recollect those incidences that gave you happiness. If you get pleasant dream in the night, you will gain energy even during sleep and you will feel fresh in the morning. If nothing is possible; count from 100 to 1 and you will sleep before you reach 1.

MENTAL BALANCE

The mind is the main source that activates the body and the vital energy in us. If the mind gets disturbed everything goes wrong. Scientifically this can be called as psychological influences. The mind is always busy even when we are sleeping. If it does not have anything to do then it starts thinking of the past, planning the future, comparing, judging and many other things. It has the habit of predicting things that this may happen or that may happen. When a person develop hatred in him for someone the mind starts thinking all negative things about him and imagines how the person should suffer. Sometime when it believes the rumour spread in the air it starts imagining the consequences that may happen to him or to the society. The mind has to be trained to remain silent when it is not engaged in any activity. Our sages and saints suggest different kinds of meditation to make the mind silent. If the mind remains silent for five minutes it has the capacity to complete the task of one hour in ten minutes. This is the approximate calculation. You could have experienced if you had a sound sleep in the night, you will feel fresh in the morning. It is because your mind remains silent throughout the night and you gained enough energy and became fresh in the morning.

The Mind cannot be kept silent without proper training. Therefore you have to take some steps to silence your mind. Meditation is one of the best method suggested by almost all the religions.

In the beginning you have to choose a place to sit for meditation where you will not be getting disturbed by other people or sources. You should select a time that you feel comfortable that you will not be worried about whether you have done this work or not.

Once you have decided the place and time, sit in a comfortable posture and close your eyes. The moment you prepare to do meditation all the thoughts that were bothering you will start coming one by one. Sometimes so many thoughts will come and disturb you at the same time. You may feel whether you have locked the door or not, what to do if my friend comes now, doubt whether your children whether they are safe or not; if you listen to a small sound, immediately the curiosity will arise to go out and see who had come viz- a- viz. You have to ignore all such thoughts; if possible you must try to understand what kinds of thoughts that are coming to you frequently when you sit for meditation. If you make an effort to ignore those thoughts, it may get away. Sometimes the thought maybe something serious that you need your attention is popping up as you are making an effort to remain silent.

In such a situation you may receive the thought and identify as to where it comes from; whether it is related to your family, friends or office. You have to go in depth to understand the problem and try to find a solution for that if possible. Once you found a solution for the thought that was disturbing, it will get away from you. This way you can minimize the number of thoughts that would help you to make your mind silent. After few days your mind will become silent when you sit for meditation. Later on, your mind will become silent at any place during given time. When your mind is silent you will be able to focus on one thought and find a solution for the same. You will be able to easily reject the unwanted thoughts entering in you from the environment.

Another way to silence the mind is to sit in a place in a given time and look at the light or the photograph of your God for a few minutes and then close your eyes with your palm for few minutes, then again repeat the same activity two or three times every day. This method will help you to find peace within you.

Another method is to chant the hymns from your Holy script or chanting the name of your God will help you to silence your mind. The hymns written by the sages and Saints contain the power in it and those who chant the hymns definitely get the positive benefit of chanting. Similarly chanting the name of the god also brings silence in the mind, peace in the heart and keeps us happy forever. Depression is a mental state that is considered as a disease. Depression is the negative result of expectation, repeated failures and deprivation of the rights. Meditation is the key to get rid of depression.

EMOTIONAL BALANCE

We normally act according to our emotions in our day to day life. When everything goes according to our wish and desire, we are happy. In case if something goes wrong, we get disappointed, we get angry, we fall in to depression and get frustrated.

In some cases, emotional disturbances results in high BP, heart attack etc. In other words emotional disturbance brings problem to our health. Therefore it becomes necessary that we should maintain emotional balance too.

Each one has around him an atmosphere made of the vibrations that come from his character, his mood, his way of thinking, feeling and acting. These atmospheres act and react on each other by contagion; the vibrations are contagious; that is to say, we readily pick up the vibrations of someone we meet, especially if that vibration is so strong. So it is easy to understand that someone who carries in and around himself peace and goodwill create the same in others. The person who enters a positive atmosphere receives at least some amount of peace and goodwill, whereas scorn, irritability and anger will arouse similar movements in others.

The next part is to deal with the people and environment with whom or where we are associated with. We will not be able to change the thoughts, feelings and activities of others but we can definitely take such measures that can help us to keep ourselves protected. Some tips with example to deal with the situation from the environment are given below:

- When a person is sick in your family and if his or her well wishers come to inquire about the health, please see to that they do not discuss any negative effect of the disease the person is suffering from. When a person is sick he needs rest; he needs peace; he needs care and love. In the name of inquiry if he is getting disturbed that will increase the amount of stress and the pressure of disease. Therefore it is necessary to keep the sick person away from the people who you come with negative kind of thoughts and feelings.

- Sometimes the sick person could have lost his hope of recovery or his opinion about the power of the disease may be very strong. In such situation, neither medicine can help nor counseling. The first thing we have to do is to make the sick person feel that he will be recovered soon. We have to give the examples of people who came out of dangerous life killing diseases. He should be made to understand that the other family members need him and he has to come out of his disease. You have to suggest him Auto Positive Suggestion method to follow. His near and dear ones can bless him to recover soon. Blessings bring wonder in others life. When you bless someone, naturally you are filled with peace and your attitude is selfless. Any selfless blessing or wish gets materialized soon.

- While preparing the food for the sick person you can say within yourself, "Let this food serve as a medicine to bring him for is recovery". These kinds of feelings performs miracle in the recovery of the person. You can do the same when you are giving the medicine to the sick person.

PRAYER

The easiest way to get rid of disease or difficulty is prayer. If the prayer is rightly done, if the faith is strong, it can cure any disease even without medicine. Let us learn how to offer our prayer so that we are always protected by the Divine grace.

Before we attempt to make any prayer, we should understand to whom we are offering our prayer; what relationship do we have with the god to whom we are asking for help. Are we sure that the God will hear our prayer and help us to come out of our problem? It is difficult to give a definite answer for this question because the faith or the belief that we have about the god is different to each individual. There are religious differences and interpretations of the religious holy scripts by different saints are also different. Each one had their own experiences and they believe that their faith is only true.

Therefore it becomes necessary to know about the God, His power, knowledge, our relationship with him etc., before submitting our prayer. According to Hindu religion the supreme Lord is the creator of the universe. He had incarnated on this earth in different forms at different times to help the human beings to understand the unconditional love.

According to Hindu mythology the time is divided into four parts. They are, Kruta Yug or Satya Yug, Treta Yug, Dwapar Yug and Kali Yug. The quality and faith of the human beings in each Yug was of similar kind.

People lived in Satya Yug were totally depending on the supreme Lord for their needs. They were truthful to each other; had unconditional love for fellow beings; performed their rituals and duties perfectly. In other words, they were like the infant in the hands of the mother. Whenever they experienced any difficulties they bowed before the God for rescue and recovery. As the mother takes care of the needs of the Infant the God also had taken care of the people who were totally dependent on him.

As the Infant grows to childhood, it tries to learn things from atmosphere, communicate to the caregiver for its needs, and tries to do things on its own. The mother loves to see the child's efforts to learn things and she also supports the child to be more independent. Similarly human beings who were totally dependent on God tried to be on their own and God has given the freedom for them to learn things. However, when the child harms himself or faces any difficulties, immediately it rushes to the mother for rescue. The mother also immediately attends to the child to solve the difficulties and make the child feel comfortable.

This is what had happened during the end of Kruta Yug. In Treta Yug Sri Ram incarnated on the earth and taught the people to live in the path of righteousness. In Treta Yug people performed spiritual rites to different form of Gods to get their problems solved. They worshiped the Fire, air, rain and planets to fulfil the requirement of their needs. In Treta Yug almost 25% of the people left the path of righteousness and engaged in demonic activities. The purpose of the incarnation of Sri Ram was to destroy the demons and protect the noble people those who trusted the God and depended on him. After the withdrawal of Sri Ram from the earth the Dwapar Yug begun.

As the child grows into adulthood, he or she becomes more independent and they would like to be with their peer group and experiment everything in life. They love to do adventures and want freedom to be independent in taking and doing anything. They find happiness in disturbing others, enjoy proving that they are the best, do anything to get recognition and want others to obey them or follow them. When the child grows into adulthood, they hide things from the parents, enter into wrong companionship and does not obey or listen to the advice of elders and parents. Therefore the parents and elders also become helpless in bringing change in the life of the adult.

Similarly when the devotees move away from the God and indulge into to evil activities and evil thoughts, the God permit them to do as they wish. In most of the cases if the demon did penance to get any boon the God appreciated the effort and the concentration of the demon and gave him the boon that he asked for.

In Dwapar Yug, 50% of the people were in the path of righteousness and 50% of the people were in the path of demonic activities. Once again the God incarnated in the form of Sri Krishna and taught the people to live in the path of righteousness. In the battlefield of Kurukshetra the teachings of Bhagavat Geeta is given by Sri Krishna to the people of Kali Yug through Arjun. He also showed the harmful effects that the evil activities bring in the life. However, those who found enjoyment in demonic or evil activities could not come back to the God and they preferred to continue in the demonic way they were living. Lord Krishna's incarnation did not go waste. Few people started understanding the teachings of the God and followed his path. And the Kaliyug started.

In Kaliyug the kingdom of Evil established its power on human beings. Anger, hatred, jealousy, revenge, fear, greed, torture, murder, falsehood and all negative qualities had been inculcated in the human beings; whereas in Treta Yug and Dwapar Yug there were few Demons and by destroying them, the incarnation of the God was able to establish the righteousness on the earth; but in Kaliyug the Asuric forces entered into the human body and every human being possesses the negative qualities in them and ultimately the love and peace which the human beings were enjoying in Kruta Yug had been disappeared. 75% of evil and 25% of noble qualities are prevailing on the earth now in Kali Yug.

The pollution of the quality of the people and the negative qualities the human beings entertain in them brings epidemic and pandemic diseases, chronic illnesses, failures and unhappiness. The only way to get rid of all these evil effects is to approach the God to come and help us in our crisis. The human being had gone far away from the God and some of them believe there is no God at all.

God helps those people who approach him. He does not demand any price for that. He wants us to be happy and let others also to be happy. God does not punish anybody for any mistakes or sins done by them, but the law of Karma brings the result for the activities done by the people in the form of thoughts words and deeds. In other words whatever the good you are enjoying in your life is the benefit of the positive things that you have done in your life and all the troubles and difficulties that comes in your life are the results of the negative things that you have done in your life.

Though the God had created the universe, he had given freedom to every living and nonliving beings and provided everything that is required for their growth, development and survival. Whether it is an insect or a plant or human beings, they were given the freedom to utilize everything that has been created by the God and in the way that gave them pleasure.

If a person utilizes the materials around him in the right way he is able to enjoy the benefit of the material; but if he had misused or wrongly used the things he faces the difficulties out of that material.

Planets & other living and non-living beings except human beings are the example for the perfect function of God's creation. All the planets are created by the supreme Lord. They function from the time unknown, but always regular in their movements. The sun never rises in the West or sets in the East. Full moon and No moon occurs once in a month. If you plant a Mango seed you get mango. Just beside the mango tree you plant an apple or orange tree. You will get apple from the apple plant and orange from the orange plant. The ground is same; the chemicals and minerals available in the earth are same; but the fruits that we get are as per the seed that are sown. The leaf, the flower and the fruits we get are different from each tree. Even the non living beings like plants and trees are given the knowledge to absorb the needed energy from the ground, from the air and from the water. A small seed turns to be a giant tree and it gives the fruits in several numbers for several years.

When a small piece of sweet falls on the ground, the ants are able to sense its food and reach there to pick up. How does an ant able to sense where it can get its food? This is the power of God that had given to an ant to understand where its food is available. We can take as many examples as required to prove the existence of God and the power of God.

Now the question comes as to who is the God. To whom we have to offer our prayer; to the Hindu God or the Christian God or the God of any other faith or religion? It is very simple. You have born in a particular religion and your parents could have guided you about the God and the methods of worshiping him. You can follow their guidance and offer your prayer to that form of God.

God is one. But his forms are many. As he has the power to create anything, destroy anything, he has the power and freedom to take birth in any form that he feels suitable for the humanity from time to time. Therefore we cannot dictate terms to God to be in a standard form or give a definition to God with our limited knowledge. You have the freedom to choose the form of the God that you feel best to offer your prayer. When God incarnated upon this earth, when he had taken human form to the human parents, naturally the parents gave him a name and brought him up. It is his love that he accepted the name given by the parents and became familiar among the people with that name.

He came as Lord Jesus, Prophet Mohammad, Mahaveer Jain, Buddha and in many other forms. In each of his incarnation he helped the people of that time to come out of evil qualities and discover the unconditional love for each other. Therefore there would be nothing wrong if you choose any form of the God to worship or to offer your prayer.

If you are too little to understand the God, the purpose of his incarnation etc., it is better to follow the guidelines given by the parents. In the meantime you must understand the presence of God in your own life to develop faith that God is there. To gain the experience of the presence of God you should to try to communicate with the God and you should experience that he is listening to you and he is answering your prayer. There are so many ways through which you can develop communication with God and you will be able to gain the experience of his love and remain under his protection at all times if you adopt any one method that are given below.

Your practice will prove you that the God is in love with you and he is with you forever and it is you who didn't recognize him earlier. Once you start developing communication with the God, automatically your negative qualities will get away from you one by one and you will develop positive and divinely atmosphere around you.

TALK TO THE GOD ON THE BED

After you lie down on the bed, but before sleeping, close your eyes and call the God in the form that you would like to talk to and imagine that the God had come to listen to you. You start your conversation from your heart (not with voice) by offering your prostration to him and request him that you would like to talk to him. Then you start your conversation by telling him your experiences on the particular day. Whatever good you have done tell him with happiness that it was his grace that helped you to do good things. Pray that you should get more such opportunities where you can do good things. Whatever wrong you have done tell him that it was your weakness and you wanted to come out of that weakness. Ask him to give you the awareness, whenever you happen to do wrong things. If someone else had hurt your feelings or you experienced any pain given by anyone, narrate the same to him and request him that you don't want the memory of that pain anymore. Forgive the person who had given you the pain and surrender the pain to the Lord. If you want to experience that the God is listening to you then you can ask him to be with you throughout the night, protect you from bad dreams, give you a peaceful sleep and ask him to wake you up at a particular time in the morning. In other words you can ask him to wake you up in such a way that you want to get up in the morning. When you wake up in the way that you asked the God, you will understand that the Lord was with you in the night and listening to what you were telling him.

When you wake up from your sleep don't jump out of your bed immediately. Close your eyes again and thank God for being with you throughout the night and listening to whatever you were telling him. In case you had peaceful sleep, dreamless sleep, you thank him for that. If you had surrendered your major problem or chronic illness, then it may take little time to get complete cure. Till such time you have to wait.

Tell the God to be with you throughout the day, to keep you happy throughout the day and help you to make others happy throughout the day. You can also tell him to help you to do good things and become aware of all evil thoughts and ideas so that you can reject them when it comes to you.

Apart from learning a method of communication to the God you also gain so many benefits given below:

- You don't get bad dreams.

- You get a peaceful sleep.

- You are able to recollect your actions and reactions during the day.

- You will be able to recognize your mistakes which you cannot do when you were involved in the activity emotionally.

- When you understand that the lord had listened to your prayer, your faith on the God becomes strong.

- When you approach the God to give away your weaknesses and develop your positive activities, the God blesses you with divinely environment that is very rare to attain.

TALK TO GOD THROUGH LETTERS

Whenever you know that you had been attacked by any disease, you can write an application to the God to relieve you from the particular disease. You can attach the doctor's prescription and report along with your letter and keep it in front of the Gods photograph where you do your prayer every day. If you want to try, after submitting the letter and the report to the God you can wait for a day or two without taking medicine and see whether you are cured or not. In case you feel that your pain is more and you want immediate relief you can keep the medicine in front of the god, request him to help you to recover immediately through the medicine and then consume the medicine. In this way, the medicine will work fast and you will recover from the illness soon.

It is not only for diseases you can write to God, but also submit your prayer to the God for any needs of yours or solution of any problem. If you keep the practice of writing your difficulties to the God and keep a record of it, it would help you to know how many times the God has helped you when you have approached him. If you are maintaining the record the letters written to the God, you should also thank him in writing whenever your prayers were answered. When you express your gratitude to the God it would do miracles in your life.

Normally we approach the God for so many things and the God listened to us and helped us several times; but human beings forget to thank the God, once the problem is solved. After sometime he forgets that it was the God who had helped him through someone or others when he was in difficulties.

The benefit of writing letter to God is that, you are able to concentrate on what you are writing. If your mind, body and vital surrender the prayer, it will work out miracle. There are so many ways to communicate to God. The doubt about the God's answer always remains in the human mind. When you select a particular method of communication to God and stick on to that method till you get the result, you will be able to understand that it is your prayer that has got you the result.

God wants to be sure as to what exactly you want. The more you are clear in your prayer for your requirement; the fast will be the result you get from the God. If you say generally, "Keep me happy. Keep me healthy", you will not know the result of your prayer. Therefore, the God sanctions such prayer which is specific, clear and with total faith. When you are not sure as to what exactly you want or when you yourself do not have the faith that you will be relieved from the illness that you are suffering from;

because of your preconceived ideas, then your prayer will not work out. When you write your prayer first think as to what exactly you want; state clearly as to what you are suffering from; in case you know the reason that it was your mistake that had caused the problem to you, accept that and ask for forgiveness.

Once you had decided that this is going to be your prayer then put the same in writing. If at all you have any doubt that the God may not help you, put that feeling also before him and accept your faithlessness. This kind of truthfulness will immediately bring the positive result. Once you had the relief from your illness, do not forget to thank him in the same method that you offered in your prayer.

GIVE YOUR BAD HABITS AND ASK THE BOON YOU WANT

We had already discussed as to how the negative qualities and negative thoughts lead us to ill health. If we have to live a healthy life we have to give up the negative habits that we are having in us.

Thinking bad about others; passing negative comments about others; not obeying the parents and elders; not doing one's duty properly; ignoring one's responsibility, finding escape for not doing the duty; unwilling to learn; overeating; less eating; oversleeping; avoiding sleep; addiction to alcohol or craving for any kind of intoxication; abusing others; harming others; indulging into verbal and physical fight; disturbing the peace of others; feeling jealousy of others achievement are some of the negative habits that every human being possess in him.

You can surrender any one of your bad habit that you feel that you can give up to the God. In return you can ask him to liberate you from any particular illness. This way you will be able to get rid of your bad habits and ultimately you will learn the art of solving your problems with the help of God. To practice this method you have to understand or list out your bad habits according to its seriousness. Thereafter you have to decide which bad habit you think you will be able to give up, because once you give up that bad habit you are not supposed to repeat it again. Similarly the bad habit that you are surrendering should be somewhat equal to what you are asking from the God. You have to justify yourself in this issue.

Mostly students those who had problem in their studies surrendered their habit of arguing or back answering to the parents and asked for knowledge in the particular subject. They were successful in getting their prayer answered.

Initially you can make simple offering for experimenting as to how this method works for you. If you are successful, this is the best way to get rid of every negative quality and enjoy the benefit of the blessings of the God and making him to be with you all the time.

CHANT THE NAME OF THE GOD AND HEAL YOURSELF

In Bhagavad Gita lord Krishna had told Arjun," If anyone takes my name at the time of his death, I will take them to my Abode even if they are the greatest sinners". Arjun replied to Sri Krishna, "It sounds very nice to hear your promise; but the fact is that we don't know when will be our death; and you had kept us in binding with the family, friends, different enjoyments etc. We are totally engrossed in our day to day life and we do not know the time of our death. How is it possible to take your name and reach you after death?" At that time Krishna advised Arjun, "You can do so by practice. If you develop the habit of calling me in your pleasures and sufferings, naturally at the time of death my name will be in your tongue".

The Lord himself had declared that he will be answering the prayer of his devotees. Chanting the name of the Lord at all circumstances will force the Lord to come to your rescue whenever you need. The more communication you have with the Lord the deep will be the relationship. God does not prescribe any particular name to chant. You are free to select the name of the God to whom you want to call, because God is one but his forms are many. While giving the statement "God Is One; But His Forms Are Many" the following example will help you.

Let us assume that your parents had given you the name "Ravi". Though you are Ravi, you will be the son for your parents, grandson to your grandparents, student to your teacher, a citizen in your country and so many other forms by which you will be recognized but the fact is that you are Ravi but people address you in different forms according to the relationship they have with you. In the same way God is one but he takes birth in human form to guide his children when they are becoming ignorant and going far away from him. People who lived during the period of the Lord's incarnation recognized him and worshipped him only in that form. Those who were not fortunate enough to be with the Lord during their lifetime, believed what the elders taught them. Since it was not their direct experience, their approach to the God was also partly mechanical partly necessity. Whenever you do anything mechanically without involvement you do not get the desired result. The reason for not receiving the answers for your prayer is either faithlessness or loss of dedication.

Whatever the religion you may belong to, you may choose a name of the God on whom you have the faith and chant his name as many times as possible throughout the day. When you are going to start a new thing you can chant the name, early in the morning when you get up you can call his name, before having your food you can call his name and offer the food to him, when you go to office instead of indulging into unwanted thoughts or unwanted things you can chant his name on the way till you reach the office. God never has any limitation when and where to chant his name. You are free to call him at any time at any place and he will be there to support you if your faith on him is strong.

Chanting the name of the god creates a positive vibration in you. The name of the Lord is considered to be Holy. Therefore chanting his name makes you pure. When the Lord understands that you are depending on him for everything and you have a relationship with him, he too will be always ready to attend to you whenever you call him. When you practically experience that the God answers your prayers and he is practically taking care of you in your life, you will feel peace, happiness and also feel comfortable in your life.

In Hindu mythology, in Ramayan, Sri Ram's devotee Sri Hanuman had to fight with his Lord Ram. Ram Baan (mystical arrow that never comes back without killing the person on home it is sent) was thrown on Hanuman to defeat him in the war. Being unable to face the arrow, Hanuman closed his eyes and started chanting the name of Ram. The arrow could not harm Hanuman because the mystical arrow was sent by Ram and it could not harm the person who chants the name of Ram. After this incident, people started saying that Ram's name is greater than Ram's Baan. There are so many spiritual evidences on the power of the name of the god in our history. Therefore to establish peace in the mind it would be better to chant the name of the god of your choice with faith and dedication.

CONCLUSION

The whole Universe is facing the challenge of the attack of Covid. Some are creating fear in the public; some are playing tricks to utilize the fear of common people and their livelihood; some are trying to mint money by illegal ways.

The fast spreading of pandemic closed down almost all the activities and created crisis in every part of life; people are coming out with their ideas to drive away Covid. If we have to put an end to this kind of pandemic and epidemic diseases, the thought of the people, and the way of looking at things should be changed. People should learn to develop positive vibration, positive environment and positive atmosphere in and around them. Self discipline to be inculcated in every human being so that they don't fall victim to desires and greediness.

This book is a step to help the people to change themselves and find a suitable method to live a disease free life.

THE END

CONCLUSION

Universe is facing that challenge of the attack of Covid. Some are creating fear in the public; some are playing tricks to utilize the fear of common people and their livelihood; indulging into selling the human body parts for the sake of money without any feeling for humanity; the spreading pandemic close down almost all the activities and created crisis in every part of life; people are coming out with their ideas to drive away Covid. The same is displayed in the YouTube without any filtration. If we have to put an end to this kind of pandemic and epidemic diseases, the thought of the people, that you have the people and the way of looking at things should be changed. Positive vibration, positive environment and positive atmosphere to be created in everyone.Self discipline to be inculcated in every human being so that they don't fall victim to desires and greediness.

This book is a step to help the people to change themselves and find a suitable method to live a disease free life.